Keto For Women Over 50

Complete Guide On How Senior Women Can Follow The Keto Diet To Lose Weight In A Healthy Way, Reset Their Hormones And Boost Their Energy

Mary Ortiz

Table of Contents

Introduction

From the time we are born, our bodies change in all aspects. For us women, the lean muscle mass already starts reducing even before we reach 50, which slows down our metabolism. Activity is reduced as a result, and less calories are burned. That leads to weight gain and this particular change is consistent even in the fitter among us.

What's more, during menopause, our hormones change and there is a significant reduction in estrogen, which creates a shift of fat to the midsection.

As a woman around this age, you might have noticed the creeping weight gain, and you might have tried a couple of things, which include cutting out a snack or moving more. However, no matter what you do, the scale never really seems to budge. This might leave you feeling stressed, worried and depressed, and wondering whether there's a better solution.

There is a solution, and this book is here to bring it to you. The solution is a diet that you might have heard of known as the ketogenic diet.

According to studies published in the *National Institutes of Health,* the ketogenic diet helps older women transition into menopause and manage the effects of this stage by resetting the estrogen and testosterone hormones, and burning the stubborn fat.

An article published in *ketodietapp.com* confirms this by asserting that the ketogenic diet balances hormones, leading to better moods, increased energy, weight loss and better overall health.

This means that if you're around 50 years old, you should lean more towards a ketogenic diet lifestyle to lose weight, feel better, increase energy and assure yourself of a good overall health. I know that it can seem daunting and challenging to start a new diet, especially if you're like most of us who don't really like dieting, but that's why this book is here.

This book will show you why the ketogenic diet is not your regular *diet*; why following it doesn't exactly feel like dieting, as well as how this diet can benefit you, how to follow the keto diet properly as a 50 year old plus, and everything else you need to know to get started the right way.

As you will find out, while the keto diet works in bringing about rapid weight loss through ketosis, the standard approach of following the diet is not exactly ideal for women over 50. You need to customize it for your age to ensure you don't end up creating more problems.

And this book will show you just that.

Let's begin with the keto basics.

against the publisher for any reparation, damages, or monetary loss due to the information herein, either directly or indirectly.

Respective authors own all copyrights not held by the publisher.

The information herein is offered for informational purposes solely, and is universal as so. The presentation of the information is without contract or any type of guarantee assurance.

The trademarks that are used are without any consent, and the publication of the trademark is without permission or backing by the trademark owner. All trademarks and brands within this book are for clarifying purposes only and are the owned by the owners themselves, not affiliated with this document.

The Basics of The Keto Diet

What Is It?

The ketogenic diet is a low carb, high fat and moderate protein diet. More specifically, it involves a fixed proportion of these three macronutrients, which is as follows:

Carbs: 5-10%

Fat: 70-75%

Protein: 20-25%

The goal of this diet is to get your body to receive lower levels of glucose you consume in form of carbohydrates, deplete the stored glucose forms of energy in the body, and therefore lead to the burning of the stored fat in the body for energy in a process referred to as ketosis.

Here's How The Diet Actually Works

As you know, the Western diets, including the Standard American diet is heavily concentrated on carbs and often leaves a small proportion to fat, if at all, as shown in the food pyramid below.

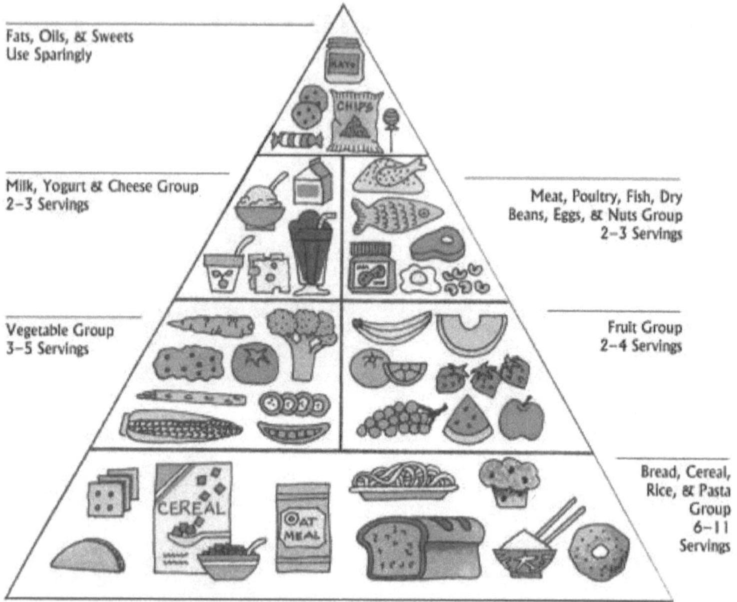

When you consume a meal that is rich in carbohydrates, you're essentially telling your body to prioritize carbs in supplying energy to the body; the body thus actively converts the carbs to glucose to use for fuel. Insulin is then secreted to carry the glucose into cells, where it is used as a source of energy.

When there is an excess of this glucose (resulting from a consistently high intake of carbs), it means your blood will consistently have high levels of insulin, this can lead to:

1.   Excessive fat storage: This happens because there is a limit to the amount of glucose body cells can accommodate. When the limit is reached, the excess glucose is stored in the liver and muscles as glycogen (conversion of glucose to glycogen takes place in the liver with the help of insulin), which also have a limit (about 2000kcal). When the glycogen stores become full, the rest of the glucose is converted to fat and stored in designated parts around the body. There's no limit to the amount of fat that can be stored.

2.   Insulin resistance (where your body is not responding to insulin effectively). This occurs when your blood is consistently flooded with insulin. This is a problem that often leads to a new host of problems, one of the major ones being an imbalanced hormonal system. In the human body, insulin is considered a major hormone, because it affects other hormones and hormone systems. This largely involves the sex hormones. This means that its state can determine the state of other hormones in the body. Therefore, during menopause, when the body is trying to

manage the effects of imbalanced hormones, having insulin resistance can worsen the problem. On the other hand, having low and stable insulin levels can influence better hormonal balance in the sex hormones in women during menopause.

Insulin resistance also disrupts fat metabolism. As we've seen, when body cells can't take in any more glucose, the glucose ends up being stored as fat. That means that at some point, when you're experiencing insulin resistance, your cells will continually be starved or glucose-deficient, even when the blood is flooded with glucose. This situation can leave you feeling exhausted all the time.

For us women who are within the menopause stage, insulin resistance can be a nightmare especially because our bodies are producing less estrogen, and one of the main functions of estrogen is to control insulin resistance.[1]

Another problem is testosterone. High levels of glucose in the body reduces the levels of testosterone. We need this hormone to maintain muscle mass, energy, bone strength

---

[1]

https://www.ncbi.nlm.nih.gov/pmc/articles/PMC4391691/

as well in weight loss. Given that this hormone reduces during menopause as well, high sugar levels in the blood makes things worse.

So obviously, having a way of managing our blood sugar levels can reduce our symptoms of menopause as the baseline by reducing weight gain, muscle loss, fatigue and the other effects of insulin resistance.

What the research says

One review published in the *National Institutes of Health* suggest that lowering your carb consumption can reduce insulin levels and increase hormonal imbalances, and as a result, make it easier to deal with menopause.[2]

Other studies published in the same website also demonstrate a correlation between insulin resistance and a higher risk of certain side effects of menopause such as hot flashes.[34]

---

[2] https://www.ncbi.nlm.nih.gov/pmc/articles/PMC5372867/

[3] https://www.ncbi.nlm.nih.gov/pmc/articles/PMC3462945/

[4] https://www.ncbi.nlm.nih.gov/pubmed/28448547

That's not all, there are certain studies that prove that reducing carb intake assists in preventing further weight gain that comes with menopause. For instance, there is one study published in *National Institutes of Health* that was conducted in more than 88,000 woman that discovered that following a good low carb diet can reduce the risk of postmenopausal weight gain.

On the other hand, following a low fat diet is associated with a high risk of weight gain.[5]

More evidence provided below.

How does the ketogenic diet help?

First, a ketogenic diet is structured to reduce carbs and increase fats, which makes it ideal in preventing weight gain as highlighted above, and improving hormonal balance during menopause and post-menopause stages.

---

[5] https://www.ncbi.nlm.nih.gov/pmc/articles/PMC5728369/

Secondly, it actively burns the already accumulated fat in the body and boosts energy.

Here's how.

The carb intake on keto is very low, and that forces the body to look for another form of energy to fuel the body cells. This is where the fats come in.

But it starts with stored glucose – in the form of glycogen.

When dietary carbs are absent or inadequate, and glucose levels in the blood are low enough (after the body has burned the available dietary glucose), the body starts breaking down the stored glucose- which in this case is the glycogen in the liver and muscle tissues.

When it gets depleted, the fats become the next target. The fats are broken down into fatty acids and glycerol, and then into ketone bodies (or ketones) which are then used by the body for energy. This last process is known as ketosis, and is the ultimate goal of the ketogenic diet.

Ketones are very powerful sources of fuel, which have been proven by science to be more efficient than glucose in providing energy throughout the body. They particularly provide sustainable energy to the brain, organs and muscles, and that's why you'll hear some experts saying that ketones are critical for human survival -since they enable the body to keep functioning at high or optimum levels even when it runs out of its natural stores (glycogen).[6]

You also need to appreciate the fact that by nature, fat digests slower than carbs. This means that when you stop eating now, you'll still receive steady amounts of energy for hours. Its quality of being a lasting energy source makes it the best source of fuel, and particularly ideal when it comes to weight loss since the body will not require "constant refilling" (as is the case with carbs).

Speaking of which, research asserts that a low-carb, high fat diet improves stability in blood glucose, which means less sugar crashes, and more stable energy.[7]

Combating cravings

During menopause, most of us tend to experience cravings and extreme hunger- especially during the transition.[8]

---

[6]

https://www.ncbi.nlm.nih.gov/pmc/articles/PMC5309297/

[7] https://www.ncbi.nlm.nih.gov/pubmed/26224300

[8] https://www.ncbi.nlm.nih.gov/pubmed/24065065

A good number of studies have proven ketogenic diet to be very effective at decreasing appetite and hunger, which could be very beneficial during menopause and post-menopause.[9]

One study that was conducted in 95 people showed that following the keto diet increases the levels of an appetite-regulating hormone referred to as glucagon-like peptide 1 (GLP-1) that is known to regulate appetite especially in women.[10]

Another small study also confirmed that a low-calorie ketogenic diet reduces appetite and levels of a hunger hormone referred to as ghrelin.[11]

---

[9] https://www.ncbi.nlm.nih.gov/pubmed/25402637

[10]
https://www.ncbi.nlm.nih.gov/pmc/articles/PMC6537934/

[11] https://www.ncbi.nlm.nih.gov/pubmed/23632752

How To Transition Into Keto In Two Steps

1. Calculate your macros and adjust gradually

As you would expect, men can decide to begin a keto diet any day and go from 300g of daily carbs in the standard American diet to 25 g without expecting major negative health effects. As women, we however require a bit more time to adjust.

Before you make any adjustment though, you need to know how much of each macronutrient you need to consume daily to lose weight and generally benefit from the keto diet, based on the standard proportion I mentioned earlier.

In case you're wondering, it is possible to go into ketosis without being specific on the figures, but for faster results, especially if you're one of those who requires a guideline, you'd need to establish the macros- even if just to ensure you don't go overboard or at least try to maintain your macro consumption within a certain range. But this can be difficult to do because there are many factors you have to consider to determine your daily macro sizes like age, body weight and level of activity. The good news is that there're many calculators you could use to get your figures right and easily.

Here's one of them:

http://bit.ly/2FtEdM7

2. Limit the carbs and increase the carbs slowly

Once you determine your daily macro sizes, the next step should be to track your regular food intake, so that you start increasing fat and reducing carbs slowly to get to those figures you determined in the previous step. This simple step will help you adopt a more conscious and deliberate approach to tracking and measuring of food in your diet.

For instance, if your target level of carb consumption per day is 50g, and you're already consuming about 250g, you can go to 150g, 100g and then 50g. The same goes for fat and protein macros. This is important to ease your hormones into a controlled and sustainable low carb lifestyle.

Check out this blueprint using the 250g mentioned above as your daily average carb consumption (but this time, with 25g as your target daily consumption amount):

- During the first week, limit your daily net calories to 150g and by the end of the week, finish this somewhere close to 100g per day.

- During the second week, begin at 100g and end the week with a daily consumption of 50g.

- By the third week, your body will be able to handle about 25g and by then, you'll have partially or fully gotten into ketosis.

Remember that for most women whose everyday lifestyle doesn't allow them to calculate and track the numbers, eating less and less carbs is the approach they often take, and it does work in many cases. It's true that the less carbs you consume, the faster you will reach ketosis but taking drastic steps may elicit negative body responses and make the process of adjusting difficult for you.

In a study that was published in the *National Institutes of Health,* 24 women who followed a low carb diet for 8 weeks lost an average of 19 pounds. They also experienced improvement in their insulin resistance, blood sugar levels as well as in the levels of triglycerides and testosterone simply by limiting their net carbs to 70g per day.[12]

This means that you don't have to target the lowest levels right off the bat to see results.

Secondly, remember that you have to listen to your body to know how long you should stay within a certain range, and how far you should reduce your carbs. For instance, if you get overly tired after getting to a certain level, you can add a few more carbs intermittently until your body is comfortable to stay within that range before you're keto or fat adapted.

Next, we will be discussing what to eat and what to avoid.

____

[12]

https://www.ncbi.nlm.nih.gov/pmc/articles/PMC4516387/

Foods To Eat And Those To Avoid

Eat This & That

To succeed with keto, you need to have a list of organic and healthy foods. Here's a good list to get you started:

Meats and seafood

- Grass-fed beef

- Fatty fish and white fish such as salmon

- Poultry like turkey and chicken

- Bacon

- Game

- Pork

- Veal

- Lamb

- Organ meats

- Sausage

- Crab

- Mussels

- Lobster

- Oysters

- Shrimp

- Octopus

- Squid

- Scallops

On the Deli counter

- Sliced chicken

- Pancetta

- Corned beef

- Roast beef

- Turkey

- Prosciutto

- Pastrami

- Ham

- Pepperoni

- Speck

- Salami

- Sliced chorizo

- Prepared chicken salad

- Egg salad

- Tuna salad

- Bologna and mortadella

- Sliced cheese

Dairy

- Heavy cream

- Butter and ghee

- Eggs

- Cheeses such as blue, brie, buffalo mozzarella, goat, Colby, gouda, Havarti, cheddar, camembert mozzarella, pepper jack, parmesan, provolone, muenster and Swiss

- Full fat crème fraiche

- Feta

- Cottage cheese

- Cream cheese

- Greek yogurt (plain)

- Ricotta

- Mascarpone

- Sour cream

- Whole milk, used sparingly

Tip: If you decide to have a meal with low fat proteins such as skinless chicken, you can add a sauce on top rather than eating plain.

But Avoid This

Cold cuts with added sugars- ensure you read the label before completing a purchase

Any meat that is pre-marinated in sugary sauces

Fats and oils

- Olive oil

- Avocado oil

- Butter

- Coconut oil

- Heavy cream

- Safflower oil (occasionally)

- Sunflower oil (occasionally)

- Corn oil (occasionally)

It's easier to limit your consumption of the last three when you avoid packaged food products in which they're often found.

Avoid

- Margarine- it contains a form of dangerous fat known as trans-fats. Among other health problems, these can lead to heart disease.

- Products with trans-fats or hydrogenated oils.

Fruits and vegetables

- Lettuce

- Greens (collard, mustard, kale, Swiss chard, spinach and turnip)

- Asparagus

- Bok choy

- Eggplant

- Celery

- Herbs,

- Mushrooms

- Rapini (broccoli raab)

- Kohlrabi

- Radishes

- Zucchini

- Tomatoes

- Artichokes

- Broccoli

- Cabbage

- Brussels sprouts

- Cucumbers

- Cauliflower

- Fennel

- Jicama

- Green beans

- Okra

- Snow peas

- Snap peas

- Turnips

- Blackberries

- Raspberries

Nuts and Seeds

- Walnuts

- Flaxseed

- Chia seeds

- Almonds

- Unsweetened nut butters (such as almond and peanut butter)

- Cashews

- Pistachios

Avoid the following:

- Sweetened nut/seed butters

- Chocolate-covered nuts

- Trail mixes containing dried fruit

Others

- Collagen Protein/ peptides

- MCT oil

- Sucralose

- Erythritol

- Xylitol

- Mitosweet

- Keto-friendly cacao nibs (check label)

Keto Diet Recipes

Breakfast

Classic Bacon And Eggs

Serves 4

Ingredients

8 eggs

Cherry tomatoes (optional)

5 ounces bacon, in slices

Fresh parsley (optional)

Directions

Set the pan over medium high heat and fry the bacon until crispy. Put on a plate and set aside. Don't discard the rendered fat.

Fry the eggs in the same pan over medium high heat by cracking them into the grease or by first cracking them into a measuring cup.

Cook the eggs however you like. To have the sunny side up, you can leave the eggs to fry on one side and cover the pan using a lid to ensure they're well cooked on top. If you want them over easy, just flip the eggs over after a couple of minutes and cook for another minute.

Cut your cherry tomatoes in half and then fry them at the same time.

Add some pepper and salt to taste.

Nutritional information per serving

Calories: 272

Net carbs: 1 g

Fat: 22 g

Protein: 15 g

Keto Chocolate Noatmeal

Serves 2

Ingredients:

1 medium head of cauliflower (equivalent to 2 1/2 cups)

1 1/2 tablespoons cacao powder

1/4 teaspoon salt

1 teaspoon – 1 tablespoon, sweetener of choice such as stevia, to taste

1 tablespoon MCT oil

4 pasture raised whole eggs, beaten

1 scoop collagen peptides

1 scoop mitosweet

Seasonal berries, unsweetened coconut or cacao nibs, to garnish (optional)

Directions

Chop the cauliflower into florets and add it to a food processor or blender. Process it until it develops a rice-like consistency.

Add the coconut milk to a wide sauce pan set over medium heat and bring to a gentle simmer.

Add the cauliflower rice and stir well until combined. Lower the heat and let the cauliflower to thicken for about 4 minutes.

Fold the beaten eggs into the pan containing the collagen powder, cacao powder, salt, mitosweet and any preferred sweetener.

Give it a gentle stir and let the eggs cook through and thicken the noatmeal. To serve, stir it again and divide it between 2 bowls.

Top it with the coconut, cacao nibs and seasonal berries.

Nutritional information per serving:

Calories: 464.9

Net Carbs: 9.7g

Total Fat: 41.2g

Protein: 22.1g

Buttery Coconut Flour Waffles

Yields 5 waffles

Ingredients

4 tablespoons coconut flour

4 tablespoons granulated stevia

2 teaspoons vanilla extract

1/2 cup butter, melted

5 eggs separate whites from yolks

1 teaspoon baking powder

3 tablespoons milk, full fat

Directions

Add the coconut flour, egg yolks, baking powder and stevia to a bowl and mix well. Add the melted butter into the mixture bit by bit, ensuring to maintain a smooth consistency.

Add the vanilla extract and milk to the butter and flour mixture and combine thoroughly.

Add the egg whites to another bowl and whisk until fluffy.

Fold spoons of the whisked egg whites gently into the flour mixture.

Add the mixture into your waffle maker and cook until it turns golden brown.

Nutritional information per serving:

Calories: 278

Net carbs: 4g

Fat: 26g

Protein: 8g

Main Course Meals (Lunch And Dinner) Recipes

Easy Shrimp Avocado Salad with Tomatoes and Feta

Serves 2

Ingredients

8 ounces of peeled and deveined shrimp, patted dry

1 small diced and drained beefsteak tomato

1/3 cup cilantro or parsley, freshly chopped

1 tablespoon lemon juice

1/4 teaspoon salt

1 large avocado diced

1/3 cup crumbled feta cheese

2 tablespoons salted butter, melted

1 tablespoon olive oil

1/4 teaspoon black pepper

Directions

Coat the shrimp with the melted butter well.

Set a pan over medium-high heat and let it heat a couple of minutes. Add the shrimp to the pan in one layer and sear for one minute or until it starts turning pink around the edges. Flip and cook until the shrimp is cooked through; this should take less than one minute.

Place the shrimp on your plate as they complete cooking, and allow them to cool as you prepare the rest of the ingredients.

Add the rest of the ingredients- including the cilantro, feta cheese, lemon juice, diced tomato, diced avocado, pepper, salt and olive oil -to a bowl, toss and mix properly.

Add the shrimp and stir properly to mix.

Add more pepper and salt to taste.

Nutritional information per serving:

Calories: 430

Net carbs: 6.5g

Fat: 33g

Protein: 24g

Herby Dry Rub Grilled Chicken

Serves 4

Ingredients

1 tablespoon fresh chopped rosemary

2 teaspoons minced garlic

1 teaspoon dried fennel seeds

Salt and pepper

1 tablespoon fresh chopped thyme

1 teaspoons whole peppercorns

8 bone-in chicken thighs

Directions

Add thyme, rosemary, peppercorns, garlic and fennel to a small bowl and combine properly. Trim the chicken with a sharp knife as desired and then season with pepper and salt.

Run the herb over the chicken, pressing it into all sides.

Put the chicken on a plate, cover and refrigerate for 2 or more hours; you can also let it chill overnight.

Get the chicken out of the fridge about 15 minutes before you start to grill.

Set the grill to medium-high heat. Apply olive oil on the grates. Put the chicken on the grill with the skin side down, and cook for about 6 minutes.

Flip the chicken to cook for 6-8 more minutes until it cooks through.

Nutritional information per serving:

Calories 275

Net Carbs 1 g

Fat 17 g

Protein 1 g

Basil, Bacon & Red Pepper Frittata

Serves 6

Ingredients

1 tablespoon olive oil

1/4 cup heavy cream

1/2 cup fresh chopped basil

9 large eggs

1 cup diced mushrooms

1 small red pepper (chopped)

Salt and pepper

8 slices bacon (chopped)

1/4 cup grated parmesan cheese

1 cup shredded mozzarella cheese

Directions

Preheat your oven to 350 degrees F.

Set your ovenproof skillet over medium-high heat and then add the oil.

When hot, cook the bacon until browned and then add in the red pepper while stirring. Cook until tender.

Crack the eggs into a medium bowl and then add the parmesan and heavy cream. Stir the mixture thoroughly to combine.

Add the mushrooms to the skillet and cook for one minute. Add the basil and a sprinkle of mozzarella cheese while stirring.

Add in the egg mixture and lift the ingredients using a spatula so that the eggs run under.

Bake for up to about 7 minutes and then broil for 5 minutes – or until it browns over the top.

Slice it and serve.

Nutritional information per serving:

Calories: 300

Net carbs: 1g

Fat: 23g

Protein: 19g

Deviled Egg Spread

Serves 16

Ingredients

10 hard-boiled large eggs

1 cup finely shredded cheddar cheese

1/4 cup finely chopped pickled banana peppers

1/4 teaspoon salt

2 teaspoons juice from pickled banana peppers

Ritz crackers and assorted fresh vegetables

1 cup miracle whip

1/2 pound cooked and crumbled bacon strips

1/4 teaspoon pepper

Directions

Add the eggs to a large bowl and whisk using a fork. Add in the whip, bacon, cheese, juice from peppers, banana peppers, pepper and salt, and stir thoroughly.

Cool until serving and when you do, serve with crackers and vegetables.

Nutrition information per serving

Calories: 149

Net Carbs: 3g

Fat: 12 g

Protein: 7 g

Roasted Cauliflower with Tahini Yogurt Sauce

Serves 4

Ingredients

1/4 cup grated Parmesan cheese

2 garlic cloves, minced

1/4 teaspoon pepper

3 tablespoons olive oil

1/4 teaspoon salt

1 small head cauliflower (roughly 1-1/2 pounds), cut into 4 wedges

<u>The sauce:</u>

1/2 cup fat-free plain Greek yogurt

1 tablespoon tahini

Dash paprika

Minced fresh parsley

1 tablespoon lemon juice

1/4 teaspoon salt

Dash cayenne pepper

Directions

Preheat your oven to 375 degrees F. Add the first five ingredients to a small bowl and mix thoroughly. Rub the mixture over the cauliflower and arrange it in a foil-lined baking pan coated with cooking spray with the cut sides facing upwards. Roast for about 45 minutes or until it turns golden brown and becomes tender.

To make the sauce, add the yoghurt, tahini, lemon juice and seasoning to a small, mix well and serve over the cauliflower.

Sprinkle with parsley and enjoy!

Nutritional information per serving:

Calories: 177

Net Carbs: 5g

Fat: 14g

Protein: 7g

Keto Zucchini Noodle Gratin

Serves 8

Ingredients

8 cups of loosely packed zucchini noodles

4 ounces of shredded gruyere cheese

3 tablespoons butter

1 cup heavy cream

<u>*Optional seasonings*</u>*:*

Fresh herbs, salt, garlic powder and pepper

Directions

Put the zucchini noodles in a mesh colander and sprinkle with salt; toss well to coat.

Let them sit over the sink for 2 or so hours. They should release a good amount of moisture. Dry and squeeze the excess moisture gently using a paper towel.

Preheat your oven to 350 degrees F and grease a 9-inch baking dish with some butter. Layer the zucchini noodles on the baking dish evenly.

Add the butter, cheese and heavy cream to a small sauce pan and combine thoroughly. Heat this mixture over medium heat until the cheese and butter melt completely and the sauce becomes smooth. Switch off the heat and add your desired seasonings.

Pour the cream over the noodles evenly and bake for roughly one hour or until the dish browns nicely. Let the mixture cook for about 15 minutes and then slice it into 8 pieces before you serve.

Nutritional information per serving:

Calories: 200

Net Carbs: 3g

Fat: 18g

Protein: 6g

Instant Pot Lemon Chicken With Garlic

Serves 6

Ingredients

1/2 teaspoon garlic powder

1/2 teaspoon red chili flakes to taste, optional

1/2 small onion chopped

Juice of 1 lemon

Zest of half a lemon

2 tablespoons heavy cream/ Coconut cream

6-8 boneless chicken thighs

Sea salt and pepper to taste

1/2 teaspoon smoked paprika

2 tablespoons olive oil

3 tablespoons butter

4 sliced or minced garlic cloves

2-4 teaspoons Italian seasoning

1/3 cup of low sodium chicken broth – you can use homemade

Chopped fresh parsley and lemon slices for garnish, if desired

Directions

Season the chicken with garlic powder, pepper, paprika, chili flakes and salt.

Set a medium skillet over medium-high heat and heat the olive oil. Cook the chicken on each side until the chicken reaches 165 degrees. Transfer the chicken to a plate and set it aside.

Return the pan to the heat and melt the butter. Stir in the garlic and onion, and then add the lemon juice to deglaze the pan and cook for one minute. Add the Italian seasoning, chicken broth and lemon zest. Add the heavy cream and arrowroot starch (if you want to have a thicker sauce).

Once the sauce bubbles and thickens up a bit, put the chicken back into the pan and let it set until hot. Add the sauce over the chicken, chop the parsley and sprinkle over it.

Serve with your favorite garnish and sides- with lemon slices if you want.

Nutritional information per serving:

Calories: 366

Net Carbs: 2g

Fat: 31g

Protein: 18 g

Snacks

Low-Carb Portabella Sliders

Yields 12 sliders

Ingredients:

1 pound grass fed beef

4 slices sharp cheddar

2 dill pickles, sliced

12 basil leaves

Salt and pepper to taste

24 baby portabella mushrooms

4 tablespoons chopped yellow onion

2 tablespoons extra virgin olive oil

Yellow mustard, sriracha, mayo or low carb ketchup (optional)

Directions

Cut off the stems from the caps of the portabella mushrooms and remove any dirt or debris with a damp paper towel.

Add 1 tablespoon olive oil to a small saucepan and heat 1 tablespoon olive oil over medium heat. Add the mushroom caps and cook for 2 minutes per side, making sure to allow the mushrooms to cook through, but retain their firmness.

Transfer the mushrooms from the pan to paper towels for the liquid to drain off.

Divide the ground beef into 12 portions, making sure to roll each one of them into a tiny disc shape. Add pepper and salt to taste. Add the rest of the olive oil to a large grill pan and heat over medium heat. When hot, add the meat and cook for 3 minutes on one side, turn and cook on the other side for the same amount of time. Cook until you're satisfied with the level of doneness achieved- you can keep it medium if you like.

Stack a burger, mushroom, cheese, pickles, onions and any condiments you like and top with another mushroom cap, and basil leaf as garnish. Insert a toothpick to hold it in place and enjoy.

Nutritional information per slider:

Calories: 267

Net carbs: 1g

Fat: 20.1g

Protein: 10.4g

Keto Cheese Roll-Ups

Serves 4

Ingredients

2 ounces butter

8 ounces cheddar cheese, edam cheese or provolone cheese in slices

Directions

Put the cheese slices on a wide chopping board

Slice the butter with a cheese slicer or cut thin pieces using a knife

Cover each slice with butter and then roll up

Serve and enjoy!

Nutritional information per serving:

Calories: 331

Net carbs: 2g

Fat: 30g

Protein: 13g

Support And Track The Process In Two Steps

1. Adopt a morning routine

As you transition into a healthier nutrition and style of eating with keto, you need to try your best to begin your morning routine by doing the following ketone enhancing activities:

- Drink a lot of water

- Take half a teaspoon of MCT oil to supplement your body's supply of fatty acids

- Take two teaspoons of coconut oil

Your ketone levels are a perfect indicator of whether your body has started utilizing the fats for energy, and to what extent. The next step below explains how you can determine progress by measuring ketones.

2. Measure your ketone levels

As you already know, being aware of your progress is important because you get to know whether to maintain the progress, improve or slow things down.

There are different ways of measuring ketones; they include:

Urine ketone strips

Results from these devices reflect the levels of ketones over the past couple of hours as opposed to the time of testing. This method is great to use if you simply want to have a rough idea of your current level of ketosis.

You can buy one on Amazon – just search Urine ketone strips

Breathalyzer

On the other hand, you can measure ketones on the breath using this device. It gives a more accurate result of ketone levels in the body compared to the urine strips. The best part about it is that it involves a single up-front cost. Once you purchase it, you'll test your ketones as often as you want.

Just like keto strips, you can find these online as well. Simply search something like 'ketosis breathalyzer testing kit' or something like that.

Blood ketone tests

You can also test your blood using more specialized devices. These will give you a more accurate method of measuring ketone levels than the aforementioned, but they're relatively expensive- especially for a person who wants to test on a regular basis.

You can buy test kits on Amazon by simply searching for "blood ketone meter".

Conclusion

We have come to the end of the book. Thank you for reading and congratulations for reading until the end.

By taking these simple steps, and particularly fine-tuning your diet as illustrated in the book, you will be able to improve your energy, lose weight, balance your hormones and generally improve your health to make your menopause and post-menopause life better and more enjoyable.

If you found the book valuable, can you recommend it to others? One way to do that is to post a review on Amazon.

Please leave a review for this book on Amazon by visiting the page below:

https://amzn.to/2VMR5qr

Thank you and good luck!

www.ingramcontent.com/pod-product-compliance
Lightning Source LLC
Chambersburg PA
CBHW051234250726
48655CB00006B/2765